The Healing Herb for Mind, Body, and Spirit

Table of Contents:

Chapter 1: Introduction

- Background of Ashwagandha

- Historical Usage and Traditional Medicine

- Modern Research and Growing Demand

Chapter 2: Botanical Profile

- Taxonomy and Classification

- Morphology and Characteristics

- Geographic Distribution

Chapter 3: Chemical Composition

- Withanolides and their Bioactivity

- Other Active Compounds

- Synergistic Effects and Therapeutic Potential

Chapter 4: Health Benefits

- Stress Reduction and Adaptogenic Properties

- Anxiety and Depression Management

- Cognitive Function and Memory Enhancement

- Immune System Support

- Anti-inflammatory and Antioxidant Effects

- Pain Management and Arthritis Relief

Chapter 5: Neuroprotective Effects

Chapter 1: Introduction

Ashwagandha, scientifically known as Withania somnifera, is a powerful herb that has been used for centuries in traditional Ayurvedic medicine. With its potent therapeutic properties and adaptogenic qualities, Ashwagandha has gained popularity worldwide as a natural remedy for various health conditions.

Background of Ashwagandha

Ashwagandha has a rich history that dates back thousands of years. It has been used in traditional Indian medicine to promote longevity, vitality, and overall well-being. In Sanskrit, "Ashwagandha" translates to "smell of the horse" due to its distinct odor and the belief that consuming it can give the strength and vitality of a horse.

Historical Usage and Traditional Medicine

Ayurvedic practitioners have long considered Ashwagandha a potent herb for balancing the body, mind, and spirit. Its adaptogenic properties have made it a staple in Ayurvedic formulations for managing stress, improving energy levels, and enhancing mental clarity. Ashwagandha has also been used to support reproductive health, boost immunity, and treat various ailments.

Modern Research and Growing Demand

In recent years, Ashwagandha has attracted attention from the scientific community, leading to numerous studies investigating its potential benefits. The research has supported traditional claims and revealed new therapeutic potentials of this incredible herb. As a result, the demand for Ashwagandha supplements and products has rapidly increased, as people recognize its value in improving overall health and well-being.

In the following chapters, we will explore the botanical profile of Ashwagandha, delve into its chemical composition, and uncover its various health benefits. Additionally, we will explore its use as a neuroprotective agent, its potential effects on cardiovascular and endocrine health, and its role in supporting sexual health and fertility. We will also discuss the safety considerations, how to incorporate Ashwagandha into your lifestyle, and its connection to holistic wellness.

Join us on this journey of discovery as we explore the world of Ashwagandha and uncover the remarkable benefits of this healing herb for the mind, body, and spirit.

Chapter 2: Botanical Profile

Taxonomy and Classification

Ashwagandha, scientifically known as Withania somnifera, belongs to the Solanaceae family, which includes other well-known plants like tomatoes and potatoes. It is a perennial shrub that can reach a height of up to five feet. The plant has small, greenish-yellow flowers and produces small, orange-red berries.

Morphology and Characteristics

Ashwagandha plants have unique morphological features. The leaves are oval-shaped, about four to six inches long, and covered with fine hairs. The roots, which are the most valued part of the plant, are thick, fleshy, and resemble a white carrot or turnip. The root's odor is often described as horse-like, hence the herb's name.

Geographic Distribution

Ashwagandha is native to the dry regions of India, Pakistan, and Sri Lanka, but it has also been introduced to other parts of the world. It thrives in arid climates and is well-adapted to sandy soil. Today, Ashwagandha is cultivated in various countries, including the United States, China, and parts of Europe, to meet the growing demand for its medicinal properties.

In the following chapters, we will explore the beneficial chemical compounds present in Ashwagandha and their pharmacological activities. We will also delve into the health benefits of Ashwagandha, including its role in stress reduction, anxiety management, cognitive function enhancement, immune system support, and its potential as an anti-inflammatory and analgesic agent. Let us unlock the secrets of this incredible herb for a healthier and balanced life.

Chapter 3: Chemical Composition

Phytochemicals in Ashwagandha

Ashwagandha contains a wide array of bioactive compounds that contribute to its medicinal properties. These phytochemicals include:

Withanolides:

Withanolides are the key

bioactive compounds in Ashwagandha. They are steroidal lactones that have been extensively studied for their various health benefits, including anti-inflammatory, antioxidant, and anti-cancer properties.

Alkaloids:

Ashwagandha contains alkaloids such as somniferine, withanine, and withasomnine, which may contribute to its sedative and anxiolytic effects.

Steroidal saponins:

These compounds, such as withanosides, have been shown to have adaptogenic and anti-stress effects.

Flavonoids:

Ashwagandha contains flavonoids like kaempferol and quercetin, which have antioxidant and anti-inflammatory properties.

Active Components and Actions

The active components of Ashwagandha interact with various biological targets in the body, leading to its therapeutic effects. Some of these actions include:

Anti-stress and Adaptogenic: Ashwagandha acts as an adaptogen, helping the body cope with stress and promoting overall well-being. It modulates the hypothalamic-pituitary-adrenal (HPA) axis and regulates the stress hormone cortisol.

Anti-inflammatory:

Ashwagandha exhibits potent anti-inflammatory properties by inhibiting pro-inflammatory cytokines and enzymes like COX-2. This action may contribute to its potential in managing inflammatory conditions.

Antioxidant:

Withanolides in Ashwagandha possess strong antioxidant activity, helping to neutralize free radicals and protect cells from oxidative damage.

Neuroprotective:

Ashwagandha has been studied for its neuroprotective effects, which may be attributed to its ability to enhance antioxidant defenses, reduce inflammation, and promote the regeneration of nerve cells.

Standardization and Quality Control

To ensure the potency and consistency of Ashwagandha products, standardization and quality control measures are crucial. Standardized extracts are typically prepared to contain a specific concentration of key bioactive compounds, such as withanolides. Quality control involves testing for purity, safety, and efficacy, ensuring that products meet established standards and specifications.

In the upcoming chapters, we will explore the wide range of health benefits associated with Ashwagandha, including its effects on stress reduction, cognitive function, immune health, and reproductive health. We will also discuss the potential side effects and precautions, as well as different forms and dosages of Ashwagandha supplementation. Aren't you excited to discover the potential of this remarkable herb? Let's dive in!

Chapter 4: Health Benefits of Ashwagandha

Stress Reduction and Anxiety Management

Ashwagandha is well-known for its ability to reduce stress and anxiety levels. Studies have shown that Ashwagandha supplementation can help lower cortisol levels, the primary stress hormone, and improve overall well-being. It has been found to enhance resilience to stress, promote relaxation, and improve sleep quality.

Cognitive Function Enhancement

Ashwagandha has been traditionally used to improve memory and enhance cognitive function. Research suggests that its antioxidant and neuroprotective properties may help protect against neurodegenerative diseases and age-related cognitive decline. The herb has also shown potential in improving attention, mental clarity, and information processing speed.

Immune System Support

Ashwagandha has immunomodulatory effects, meaning it can help balance and support the immune system. It has been found to increase the activity of natural killer cells and promote the production of antibodies, enhancing the body's defense against infections. Ashwagandha supplementation may also help reduce inflammation and support overall immune health.

Anti-Inflammatory and Analgesic Properties

Withanolides and other compounds present in Ashwagandha have demonstrated significant anti-inflammatory effects. They inhibit the activity of pro-inflammatory cytokines and enzymes, thereby reducing inflammation in the body. This anti-inflammatory action may also contribute to Ashwagandha's potential as an analgesic or pain-relieving agent.

Reproductive Health and Fertility

Ashwagandha has been traditionally used to support reproductive health, particularly in men. It has been found to improve semen quality, increase sperm count and motility, and enhance testosterone levels. In women, Ashwagandha supplementation may help regulate menstrual cycles and improve fertility.

These are just a few of the many potential health benefits associated with Ashwagandha. As we uncover more information in the upcoming chapters, you will gain a deeper understanding of how this herb can positively impact your health and well-being. Stay tuned for more fascinating insights!

Chapter 5: Ashwagandha's Effect on Stress and Anxiety Disorders

Generalized Anxiety Disorder (GAD)

Ashwagandha has been studied for its potential to alleviate symptoms of generalized anxiety disorder (GAD). Several clinical trials have shown that Ashwagandha supplementation can reduce anxiety levels and improve overall well-being in individuals with GAD. It is believed to work by modulating neurotransmitters and reducing the activity of the stress response system.

Social Anxiety Disorder (SAD)

Social anxiety disorder, also known as social phobia, is characterized by intense fear and anxiety in social situations. Preliminary studies suggest that Ashwagandha may have a positive impact on reducing social anxiety symptoms. It has been found to enhance social functioning, reduce self-consciousness, and improve overall quality of life in individuals with social anxiety disorder.

Post-Traumatic Stress Disorder (PTSD)

Post-traumatic stress disorder (PTSD) is a mental health condition that develops after experiencing or witnessing a traumatic event. Ashwagandha has shown promise in alleviating symptoms associated with PTSD. Research suggests that it helps reduce anxiety, hyperarousal, and intrusive thoughts commonly experienced by individuals with PTSD.

Stress-Related Insomnia

Stressors can often lead to sleep disturbances and insomnia. Ashwagandha has been found to promote relaxation and improve sleep quality, making it potentially beneficial for individuals with stress-related insomnia. It may help reduce the time it takes to fall asleep, increase total sleep time, and improve overall sleep efficiency.

Stress Management and Overall Well-being

Ashwagandha is widely regarded as an adaptogen, a class of herbs that help the body adapt to stress and promote balance. By reducing cortisol levels and improving resilience to stress, Ashwagandha supplementation can have a positive impact on overall well-being. It may help improve mood, enhance concentration, and promote a sense of calm and relaxation.

The potential of Ashwagandha in managing stress and anxiety disorders is promising, but it is important to note that further research is needed to fully understand its mechanisms of action and determine optimal dosages. Consult with a healthcare professional before starting any supplementation regimen for mental health conditions.

Chapter 6: Ashwagandha and its Antioxidant Properties

Understanding Oxidative Stress

Oxidative stress occurs when there is an imbalance between the production of reactive oxygen species (ROS) and the body's ability to detoxify them or repair the resulting damage. This imbalance can lead to cellular damage, inflammation, and the development of various diseases. Antioxidants play a crucial role in neutralizing these harmful ROS and protecting the body from oxidative stress.

Ashwagandha's Antioxidant Compounds

Ashwagandha is rich in antioxidants, including flavonoids, tannins, phenolic compounds, and withanolides. These compounds have been shown to scavenge free radicals and inhibit oxidative damage. Withanolides, in particular, have demonstrated potent antioxidant activity and have been extensively studied for their health-promoting effects.

Protection against Chronic Diseases

By reducing oxidative stress, Ashwagandha may help protect against the development of chronic diseases. Research suggests that its antioxidant properties may play a role in preventing conditions such as cardiovascular disease, neurodegenerative disorders, cancer, diabetes, and autoimmune diseases. Ashwagandha's ability to combat inflammation and modulate the immune system further contributes to its potential in disease prevention.

Anti-Aging Effects

Oxidative stress is a major contributor to the aging process. Ashwagandha's antioxidant compounds can help neutralize free radicals and reduce the damage caused by oxidative stress, potentially slowing down the aging process. Studies have indicated that Ashwagandha can promote the production of collagen, improve skin elasticity, and reduce the appearance of wrinkles and fine lines.

Neuroprotective Effects

The brain is highly susceptible to oxidative damage due to its high metabolic activity and relatively low antioxidant defenses. Ashwagandha's antioxidant properties can help protect brain cells from oxidative stress and reduce the risk of neurodegenerative diseases. Research suggests that Ashwagandha may play a role in improving memory, cognition, and overall brain health.

Enhancing the Body's Antioxidant Defense System

In addition to its direct antioxidant effects, Ashwagandha has been found to enhance the body's own antioxidant defense system. It can increase the activity of antioxidant enzymes, such as superoxide dismutase (SOD) and catalase, thus providing a further boost in combating oxidative stress.

As we delve deeper into the research surrounding Ashwagandha, we discover the multitude of ways this ancient herb can support our health and well-being. The next chapter will explore its potential benefits for physical performance and muscle strength.

Chapter 7: Ashwagandha and Physical Performance

Understanding Physical Performance

Physical performance refers to an individual's ability to perform physical tasks, such as exercise, sports, or other physical activities. It involves factors such as strength, endurance, speed, agility, and overall fitness. Many individuals seek ways to optimize their physical performance, whether it be for athletic competitions or simply for maintaining a healthy and active lifestyle.

Ashwagandha and Strength Enhancement

Ashwagandha has long been used in traditional medicine as a natural remedy for increasing strength and vitality. Several studies have investigated its potential benefits for improving muscle strength and power. Research suggests that Ashwagandha supplementation may lead to increased muscle mass, enhanced muscular strength, and improved muscle recovery following exercise.

Endurance and Stamina Boosting Effects

In addition to strength enhancement, Ashwagandha may also have positive effects on endurance and stamina. By reducing exercise-induced stress and supporting optimal energy utilization, Ashwagandha supplementation has been shown to increase endurance levels during physical activities. This could be particularly beneficial for athletes or individuals engaging in prolonged exercise.

Stress Reduction and Exercise Performance

Exercise-induced stress can negatively impact physical performance and recovery. Ashwagandha's adaptogenic properties help the body adapt to physical stressors and reduce the release of stress hormones. This can lead to improved exercise performance, reduced exercise-induced fatigue, and faster recovery times.

Testosterone and Hormonal Balance

Ashwagandha has been found to have positive effects on hormonal balance, including the regulation of testosterone levels. Testosterone plays a crucial role in muscle growth, strength development, and overall physical performance. Ashwagandha supplementation has been shown to increase testosterone levels in men, which may contribute to improved physical performance.

Combating Inflammation and Exercise-Induced Muscle Damage

Intense exercise can generate inflammation and cause muscle damage. Ashwagandha's anti-inflammatory properties and antioxidant compounds can help reduce exercise-induced inflammation and protect against muscle damage. This may result in faster recovery, reduced muscle soreness, and improved overall performance.

Ashwagandha and Athletic Performance

The combination of Ashwagandha's various benefits, including enhanced strength, endurance, stress reduction, and hormonal balance, makes it a promising natural supplement for improving athletic performance. Whether it be for professional athletes or individuals engaged in regular physical activities, Ashwagandha may provide a natural and effective means of enhancing physical performance.

In the next chapter, we will explore Ashwagandha's potential benefits for managing stress and promoting mental well-being.

Chapter 8: Ashwagandha and Stress Management

Understanding Stress

Stress is a normal physiological response that occurs when an individual experiences pressure or demand that exceeds their ability to cope. While some stress can be beneficial, chronic stress can have detrimental effects on both physical and mental health. Managing stress is crucial for overall well-being.

Ashwagandha as an Adaptogen

Ashwagandha is classified as an adaptogen, a natural substance that helps the body adapt to and resist various stressors. It works by regulating the body's stress response systems, including the hypothalamic-pituitary-adrenal (HPA) axis and the sympathetic nervous system. Ashwagandha's adaptogenic properties make it a potential tool for managing stress.

Reducing Stress Hormones

Stress activates the release of stress hormones like cortisol and adrenaline, which can contribute to various negative health effects when chronically elevated. Research suggests that Ashwagandha supplementation can reduce cortisol levels, helping to alleviate the physiological effects of stress and promote a sense of calmness.

Improving Mood and Mental Well-being

Chronic stress can negatively impact mood and mental well-being, leading to anxiety, depression, and other mental health issues. Ashwagandha has been shown to have anxiolytic and mood-enhancing effects, potentially alleviating symptoms of stress-related mental disorders.

Enhancing Cognitive Function

Stress can impair cognitive function, including memory, focus, and decision-making. Ashwagandha may have neuroprotective effects and promote brain health by reducing oxidative stress and inflammation, which can contribute to improved cognitive function and mental clarity.

Sleep Quality and Stress Reduction

Stress can disrupt sleep patterns and contribute to insomnia or poor sleep quality. Ashwagandha has been found to have sedative properties and promote restful sleep. By reducing stress and anxiety, Ashwagandha supplementation may contribute to better sleep quality and overall restfulness.

Combating Fatigue and Boosting Energy

Chronic stress can contribute to fatigue and low energy levels. Ashwagandha's adaptogenic properties may help combat fatigue by reducing stress-induced exhaustion and promoting healthy energy levels. This can lead to improved physical and mental performance.

Ashwagandha and Overall Well-being

By managing stress and promoting mental well-being, Ashwagandha can contribute to overall health and quality of life. Whether it be combating work-related stress, improving mood, or enhancing cognitive function, Ashwagandha offers a natural and holistic approach to stress management.

In the next chapter, we will explore Ashwagandha's potential benefits for enhancing immune function and supporting overall immune health.

Chapter 9: Ashwagandha and Immune Health

Understanding the Immune System

The immune system plays a vital role in protecting the body against infections and diseases. It consists of a complex network of cells, tissues, and organs that work together to identify and eliminate foreign invaders. Maintaining a strong and balanced immune system is crucial for optimal health.

Ashwagandha's Immunomodulatory Effects

Research suggests that Ashwagandha has immunomodulatory properties, meaning it can help regulate and balance the immune system. It has been found to increase the activity of certain immune cells, such as natural killer cells and macrophages, which play a crucial role in fighting off infections.

Boosting Immune Function

Ashwagandha's ability to enhance immune function makes it a potential tool for boosting overall immunity. It has been shown to increase the production of antibodies, improve the ability of immune cells to engulf and destroy pathogens, and stimulate the release of cytokines, which regulate immune responses.

Anti-inflammatory Effects

Chronic inflammation can weaken the immune system and contribute to the development of various diseases. Ashwagandha has been found to have anti-inflammatory properties, potentially reducing inflammation and supporting a healthier immune response.

Stress and Immune Function

Stress can have a negative impact on the immune system, making individuals more susceptible to infections and diseases. As an adaptogen, Ashwagandha can help reduce stress and normalize stress hormone levels, thereby indirectly supporting immune function.

Supporting Respiratory Health

Respiratory infections, such as the common cold and flu, are common and can be challenging to manage. Ashwagandha has been found to have antimicrobial properties against certain respiratory pathogens, potentially supporting respiratory health and reducing the risk of infections.

Potential Use in Autoimmune Disorders

Autoimmune disorders occur when the immune system mistakenly attacks healthy cells and tissues. While further research is needed, some studies suggest that Ashwagandha's immunomodulatory effects may help regulate immune responses and alleviate symptoms associated with autoimmune disorders.

Ashwagandha and Overall Well-being

By supporting immune health and reducing inflammation, Ashwagandha can contribute to overall well-being and resilience against common infections. It offers a natural and holistic approach to immune support, allowing individuals to maintain a healthy and robust immune system.

In the next chapter, we will explore the potential benefits of Ashwagandha for athletic performance and recovery.

Chapter 10: Ashwagandha for Athletic Performance and Recovery

Importance of Athletic Performance and Recovery

Athletic performance and recovery are essential for athletes and individuals engaged in physical activities. Improving performance and enhancing recovery time can optimize training outcomes and help prevent injuries.

Ashwagandha's Adaptogenic Properties

Ashwagandha is widely recognized for its adaptogenic properties, which can help the body cope with physical and mental stress. This makes it a valuable tool for athletes looking to improve their performance and recover more effectively.

Enhancing Physical Performance

Research suggests that Ashwagandha supplementation may have a positive impact on physical performance. It has been found to increase muscle strength, power, and endurance, thereby improving overall athletic performance.

Supporting Muscle Recovery

Intense physical activity can lead to muscle damage and inflammation. Ashwagandha has been shown to possess anti-inflammatory properties, helping to reduce exercise-induced muscle damage and promote faster recovery.

Reducing Exercise-Induced Stress

Intense exercise can trigger oxidative stress and inflammation in the body. Ashwagandha's antioxidant and anti-inflammatory properties may help reduce exercise-induced stress, minimizing the risk of fatigue and enhancing recovery.

Enhancing Endurance and Stamina

Ashwagandha supplementation has been studied for its potential to improve endurance and stamina. It may enhance oxygen utilization, increase aerobic capacity, and delay the onset of fatigue, making it valuable for endurance-based athletes.

Supporting Hormonal Balance

Ashwagandha has been found to influence hormone levels, including cortisol, a hormone associated with stress. By helping to balance hormone levels, Ashwagandha may contribute to better recovery and performance.

Mental Clarity and Focus

Athletic performance is not just dependent on physical capabilities but also mental clarity and focus. Ashwagandha's adaptogenic properties may help reduce stress, improve sleep quality, and enhance cognitive function, positively impacting performance.

Combating Exercise-Induced Insomnia

Intense exercise can disrupt sleep patterns, leading to sleep disturbances and insomnia. Ashwagandha may help promote restful sleep and combat exercise-induced insomnia, allowing for proper recovery.

Using Ashwagandha as a Sports Supplement

Ashwagandha can be used as a natural sports supplement to support athletic performance and recovery. It can be taken in various forms, including capsules, powders, or tinctures, preferably under the guidance of a healthcare professional or sports nutritionist.

In the next chapter, we will explore the potential benefits of Ashwagandha for mental health and well-being.

Chapter 11: Ashwagandha for Mental Health and Well-being

The Impact of Mental Health on Overall Well-being Mental health plays a crucial role in our overall well-being. Poor mental health can lead to various conditions like anxiety, depression, and stress, affecting our quality of life. It is essential to prioritize mental well-being for a balanced and fulfilling life.

Ashwagandha's Adaptogenic Properties for Stress Reduction Ashwagandha has long been used in Ayurvedic medicine for its stress-reducing properties. Its adaptogenic nature helps the body adapt to stress and may help reduce symptoms of anxiety and depression.

Managing Anxiety and Depression

Research suggests that Ashwagandha supplementation may have a positive impact on anxiety and depression symptoms. It may help reduce stress levels, support a healthy mood, and improve overall mental well-being.

Enhancing Cognitive Function

Ashwagandha has been studied for its potential cognitive-enhancing effects. It may improve memory, attention, and information processing speed, thereby supporting healthy brain function and mental clarity.

Promoting Sleep Quality

Sleep disturbances can significantly affect mental health. Ashwagandha's calming properties may help improve sleep quality by reducing stress and promoting relaxation, aiding in overall mental well-being.

Supporting Neuroprotection

Ashwagandha has been found to possess neuroprotective properties, which means it may help protect brain cells from damage. This could have long-term benefits for mental health and overall cognitive function.

Boosting Energy and Vitality

Chronic fatigue and low energy levels can negatively impact mental health. Ashwagandha's ability to reduce stress and support adrenal function may help boost energy levels, promoting a more positive mental state.

Enhancing Social Functioning

Ashwagandha's ability to reduce stress and anxiety may have positive effects on social functioning. It may help individuals feel more at ease in social situations, improving overall mental well-being.

Combining Ashwagandha with Other Therapies Ashwagandha can be used as a complementary therapy alongside other mental health treatments. However, it is important to consult with a healthcare professional before incorporating Ashwagandha into a treatment plan.

The Future of Ashwagandha in Mental Health

As scientific research on Ashwagandha continues to grow, its potential benefits for mental health are becoming more prominent. Further studies are needed to explore its mechanisms of action and efficacy, paving the way for its integration into mental health treatments.

In the next chapter, we will conclude the book and summarize the key takeaways from our exploration of Ashwagandha's potential benefits for overall health and well-being.

Chapter 12: Conclusion and Key Takeaways

Summary of Ashwagandha's Benefits

Throughout this book, we have explored the various potential benefits of Ashwagandha for overall health and well-being. From its adaptogenic properties for stress reduction to its potential positive effects on mental health, cognitive function, sleep quality, and energy levels, Ashwagandha offers a holistic approach to improving our quality of life.

The Importance of Evidence-Based Research

While traditional Ayurvedic medicine has long valued Ashwagandha for its therapeutic properties, it is essential to rely on evidence-based research to understand its true potential and efficacy. Scientific studies provide us with valuable insights into how Ashwagandha interacts with the body and its potential benefits.

Consulting with Healthcare Professionals

Before incorporating Ashwagandha into your healthcare regimen, it is crucial to consult with a healthcare professional. They can provide personalized guidance based on your specific health needs and considerations.

Understanding Potential Side Effects and Interactions like any other supplement or medication

Ashwagandha may have potential side effects and interactions. It is important to be aware of these and discuss them with your healthcare professional to ensure safe and effective use.

Individual Variations and Responses

It is worth noting that each individual's response to Ashwagandha may vary. Factors such as dosage, duration of use, and individual health conditions can influence the outcomes. Regular monitoring and open communication with a healthcare professional can help optimize your experience.

Integrating Ashwagandha into a Healthy Lifestyle

Ashwagandha is not a magic solution but rather a tool that can complement a holistic approach to health. Incorporate Ashwagandha as part of a healthy lifestyle that includes a balanced diet, regular exercise, adequate sleep, stress management techniques, and other beneficial habits.

The Potential of Ashwagandha for Further Research

While Ashwagandha shows promise in various areas of health, there is still much to learn. Continued research can help uncover its full potential, including its mechanisms of action, optimal dosages, and potential applications in different health conditions.

Final Thoughts

Ashwagandha, with its rich history and potential benefits, offers a natural and holistic approach to improving our overall health and well-being. By understanding the evidence behind its potential therapeutic effects and responsibly integrating it into our lives, we can enhance our journey towards optimal health and vitality.

Thank you for joining us on this exploration of Ashwagandha, and we hope this book has provided you with valuable insights and knowledge.

Chapter 13: Frequently Asked Questions about Ashwagandha

In this chapter, we will address some common questions that people may have about Ashwagandha and its use. These questions cover a wide range of topics and can help provide clarity and additional information.

Is Ashwagandha safe for everyone to use?

Ashwagandha is generally considered safe for most individuals when taken within the recommended dosage range. However, specific populations, such as pregnant or breastfeeding women, individuals with certain medical conditions, or those taking certain medications, should consult with their healthcare professional before using Ashwagandha.

Can Ashwagandha help with weight loss?

While Ashwagandha has not been specifically studied for weight loss purposes, it may indirectly contribute to weight management by reducing stress levels, improving sleep quality, and increasing energy levels. These factors can support efforts towards a healthy lifestyle, which is essential for long-term weight management.

Is Ashwagandha addictive?

No, Ashwagandha is not addictive. It is a natural herb and does not contain addictive substances. However, it is important to use Ashwagandha within the recommended dosage range and to consult with a healthcare professional for personalized guidance.

How long does it take for Ashwagandha to work?

The time it takes for Ashwagandha to work can vary from person to person. Some individuals may experience noticeable benefits within a few weeks, while others may take longer. Consistency and regular use are key, as Ashwagandha's effects may accumulate over time.

Can I take Ashwagandha alongside other medications or supplements?

It is important to talk to your healthcare professional before taking Ashwagandha alongside other medications or supplements. They can provide guidance on potential interactions and help you make an informed decision.

Can Ashwagandha be used as a substitute for medication?

Ashwagandha should not be used as a substitute for prescribed medication without consulting with a healthcare professional. It can be used as a complementary tool to support overall well-being but should not replace necessary medical treatments.

Can I take Ashwagandha for a specific health condition?

Ashwagandha is not intended to treat, diagnose, or cure specific health conditions. However, some research suggests its potential benefits for certain conditions. It is important to consult with a healthcare professional to determine if Ashwagandha may be suitable for your specific health needs.

How should I choose an Ashwagandha supplement?

When choosing an Ashwagandha supplement, look for reputable brands that use high-quality ingredients and have undergone third-party testing for purity and potency. It is also essential to check the dosage and ensure it aligns with your specific health goals and needs.

These answers can provide general guidance, but individual circumstances and health factors may vary. It is always best to consult with a healthcare professional for personalized advice and guidance when considering the use of Ashwagandha.

Chapter 14: Tips for Incorporating Ashwagandha into Your Daily Routine

In this chapter, we will provide some practical tips for incorporating Ashwagandha into your daily routine to maximize its benefits and make it a seamless part of your wellness regimen.

Start with the recommended dosage

It is important to start with the recommended dosage of Ashwagandha and gradually increase it if needed. The optimal dosage can vary depending on various factors, including your age, weight, and health condition. Consulting with a healthcare professional can help determine the right dosage for you.

Choose the right form

Ashwagandha can be found in various forms, including capsules, powders, and liquid extracts. Choose the form that is most convenient and comfortable for you. Capsules are typically easy to take and can be incorporated into your daily supplement routine. Powders can be mixed into smoothies, juices, or other beverages, while liquid extracts can be added to water or other liquids.

Consider taking Ashwagandha with a meal

While Ashwagandha can generally be taken with or without food, taking it with a meal can help with absorption and reduce the likelihood of any stomach discomfort. Additionally, combining Ashwagandha with a meal that contains healthy fats may enhance its absorption as it is fat-soluble.

Be consistent in your usage

To experience the full benefits of Ashwagandha, it is important to be consistent in your usage. Incorporate it into your daily routine and take it at the same time each day. This helps maintain steady levels of Ashwagandha in your system and allows for optimal results over time.

Consider combining Ashwagandha with other adaptogens

Ashwagandha belongs to a group of herbs known as adaptogens, which help the body adapt to stress. Consider combining Ashwagandha with other adaptogenic herbs like Rhodiola, Ginseng, or Holy Basil to enhance its stress-reducing effects. Just ensure that you consult with a healthcare professional about the appropriate dosage and potential interactions.

Listen to your body

Everyone's body responds differently to Ashwagandha. Pay attention to how you feel before and after incorporating it into your routine. Observe any changes in your stress levels, energy, sleep quality, or overall well-being. This self-awareness can help you determine the right dosage and the optimal time to take Ashwagandha for maximum benefits.

Maintain a healthy lifestyle

While Ashwagandha can provide support for various aspects of health, it is important to remember that it is not a magic bullet. To experience its full potential, maintain a healthy lifestyle alongside taking Ashwagandha. This includes following a balanced diet, engaging in regular physical activity, getting enough sleep, and managing stress through relaxation techniques or practices like meditation or yoga.

By incorporating these tips into your daily routine, you can optimize the benefits of Ashwagandha and support your overall well-being. Remember to consult with a healthcare professional before starting any new supplement regimen to ensure it aligns with your individual needs and health goals.

This book is dedicated to all those seeking to improve their well-being and find balance in their lives.

To those who are on a journey of self-discovery and self-care, may this book serve as a guide and a source of inspiration.

To the individuals who have embraced the power of nature's gifts and are open to exploring the benefits of Ashwagandha, may this book provide valuable insights and practical tips for incorporating this ancient herb into your daily routine.

To the healthcare professionals and experts who have dedicated their lives to holistic wellness, thank you for sharing your knowledge and expertise, and for helping others find harmony and vitality.

And finally, to my loved ones, friends, and family, thank you for your unwavering support and encouragement. Your presence in my life is a constant reminder of the importance of well-being and the need to take care of ourselves and each other.

May this book bring comfort, guidance, and a renewed sense of wellness to all who read it.

With gratitude,

Charles Gayton III